PREGNANCY COMPASS

for a FIRST-TIME MOM

Everything You Need to Know about Your Baby's Growth and Development, Your Body Changes and Your Prenatal Care Options

Harbbie Yeenks

Copyright

CONTENT

INTRODUCTION

Welcome to "Pregnancy Compass: Everything You Need to Know About Your Baby's Growth and Development, Your Body Changes, and Your Prenatal Care Options." Congratulations on going on the great adventure of becoming a mommy! As a first-time parent myself, I understand the combination of excitement, pleasure, and often overwhelming feelings that come with pregnancy. That's why I developed this book — to equip you with the information, support, and direction you need to navigate this transforming event with confidence.

My path into parenthood was a whirlwind of emotions and learning experiences. From the time I realised I was pregnant, I was thrilled with a feeling of surprise and anticipation. But I also had innumerable questions and worries. I searched out reputable information, connected with other parents, and learned from experts, all in an attempt to comprehend what was happening to my body and how to best care for my developing kid.

Through my own experiences and significant study, I concluded that there was a need for a comprehensive resource that would empower first-time parents like you. And that's why I created "Pregnancy Compass." This book is your trusted companion, giving you a roadmap to traverse the many phases of pregnancy and educating you to make educated choices for yourself and your baby.

*Here are three convincing reasons why you should acquire **"Pregnancy Compass"** and make it an integral part of your prenatal journey:*

1. Comprehensive and Reliable Information: "Pregnancy Compass" is a comprehensive reference that covers all you need to know about your baby's growth and development, your bodily changes, and your prenatal care alternatives. It is painstakingly researched and written in a straightforward and accessible way, ensuring that you have accurate and up-to-date information at your fingertips. From comprehending the phases of fetal growth to learning about prenatal testing and screenings, this book delivers a wealth of information to empower you during your pregnancy.

2. Personal Experience and Empathy: As a first-time parent myself, I understand the particular difficulties and emotions that accompany pregnancy. In "Pregnancy Compass," I offer my own personal experiences, stories, and observations, building a relationship with you as a reader. This relatability and empathy will help you feel understood and supported as you navigate the ups and downs of this transforming journey. You may trust that the counsel and information presented in this book come from someone who has gone through it all.

Practical ideas and guidance: "Pregnancy Compass" goes beyond theoretical information and gives you practical ideas and guidance to manage the many elements of pregnancy. From self-care practices to diet and exercise advice, this book gives tangible actions that you may adopt in your everyday life.

You'll also receive assistance in making a birth plan, understanding pain treatment choices throughout labour, and caring for your infant during the postpartum period. These practical insights will empower you with the skills you need to make educated choices and proudly embrace parenting.

By buying "Pregnancy Compass," you are not only investing in a book – you are investing in your well-being and the well-being of your kid. This thorough book will be your valued companion throughout your pregnancy journey, giving you the information, support, and direction you need to manage this transforming event with confidence.

So, whether you are just beginning your pregnancy adventure or reaching the finish, "Pregnancy Compass" is here to help you every step of the way.

I encourage you to engage in this changing journey with me, and I am thrilled to be a part of your pregnancy experience.

Are you ready to tackle pregnancy with confidence? Purchase "Pregnancy Compass" now and empower yourself with the information and support you need to embrace this beautiful adventure.

Chapter 1

THE FIRST
TRIMESTER

Bringing a new life into the world is a wonderfully remarkable and awe-inspiring event. From the time of conception until the delivery of your wonderful baby, pregnancy is a journey filled with wonder, anticipation, and change. In this chapter, we will dig into the extraordinary process of pregnancy, concentrating primarily on the first trimester. This vital phase lays the groundwork for your baby's growth and brings about substantial changes in your body and emotions.

Physical and Emotional Changes

The first trimester is a period of tremendous physical and emotional changes as your body prepares to nourish and support the developing life inside you. Hormonal variations are responsible for many of these alterations. You may suffer breast soreness, exhaustion, frequent urination, and morning sickness, which may vary from moderate nausea to continuous vomiting. These symptoms are typically accompanied by mood swings, heightened emotions, and a sensation of exhilaration mixed with worry. It is crucial to note that every woman's experience is unique, and although some may have an easy first trimester, others may have more obstacles. It is vital to seek help from your healthcare practitioner and loved ones at this time.

Stages of Fetal Development and Growth

During the first trimester, your baby experiences fast development and growth. It is genuinely awe-inspiring to see the change from a small collection of cells to a recognizable human form. Let's investigate the phases of fetal development:

The Germinal Stage

The germinal stage is the very beginning of pregnancy and lasts from the time of fertilization until roughly two weeks. It begins when the sperm fertilizes the egg, resulting in the development of a single-celled zygote. The zygote then experiences fast cell division as it moves down the fallopian tube towards the uterus. Around the fifth day following fertilization, the zygote inserts itself into the uterine lining, a process termed implantation. This signals the conclusion of the germinal stage and the beginning of the embryonic stage.

The Embryonic Stage

The embryonic stage covers from the implantation of the zygote, about week 3, until the conclusion of the eighth week. During this time, the embryo establishes the foundations of key organs, bodily systems, and external traits.

At the beginning of the embryonic stage, the cells quickly divide and differentiate into three separate layers: the ectoderm, mesoderm, and endoderm. Each layer gives birth to distinct organs and tissues. The ectoderm develops into the nervous system, skin, hair, and nails. The mesoderm creates the muscles, bones, heart, kidneys, and reproductive organs. The endoderm gives birth to the respiratory system, digestive system, liver, and pancreas.

Around week four, the neural tube begins to develop from the ectoderm. This structure ultimately forms the brain and spinal cord. The heart also begins to beat, and the circulatory system starts to form, enabling the transfer of oxygen and nutrients to the growing embryo.

By the conclusion of the embryonic stage, the embryo is about one inch long and is now referred to as a fetus. Basic facial characteristics, including the eyes, nose, and mouth, start to take form. The limb buds sprout, which will ultimately grow into arms and legs. The primary organs continue to grow and become increasingly specialized. The placenta also develops at this period and performs a key function in supplying oxygen and nutrition to the baby and removing waste products.

How the Placenta Aids the Growth of the Fetus During the Embryonic Stage

During the embryonic stage, the placenta performs a key function in supporting the growth of the fetus. The placenta is an organ that originates in the uterus and functions as a contact between the mother and the growing embryo/fetus. It serves crucial functions that are necessary for the development and well-being of the growing newborn. Here's how the placenta aids fetal development throughout the embryonic stage:

• Nutrient and Oxygen Supply

The placenta enables the flow of nutrients and oxygen from the mother's circulation to the growing baby. The mother's blood, bringing oxygen and nutrients, passes via the placenta, which includes a network of blood arteries called chorionic villi. These designs enhance the surface area accessible for exchange. Oxygen and nutrients, such as glucose and amino acids, flow from the mother's blood via the placenta's villi and into the fetal circulation. This ensures that the growing embryo/fetus obtains the essential nutrients for growth and development.

• Waste Elimination

The placenta also assists in eliminating waste items created by the growing embryo/fetus. Carbon dioxide and other waste products are transferred from the fetal circulation to the mother's bloodstream via the placenta. The maternal circulation takes these waste products away from the growing infant and removes them via the mother's excretory organs, such as the lungs and kidneys.

• Hormone Production

The placenta generates hormones that are crucial for sustaining pregnancy and promoting fetal growth. One of the most essential hormones generated by the placenta is human chorionic gonadotropin (hCG). HCG helps maintain the synthesis of hormones, including estrogen and progesterone, which are vital for prolonging the pregnancy. These hormones serve a key role in encouraging the development of the uterus, maintaining the uterine lining, and delaying menstruation.

• Immune Protection

The placenta works as a barrier, sheltering the growing fetus from the mother's immune system. The mother's immune cells are kept from attacking the growing embryo/fetus by numerous processes, including the development of specific cells and chemicals inside the placenta. This permits the fetus to grow without being rejected by the mother's immune system.

• Endocrine Function

In addition to hormone synthesis, the placenta also has endocrine functions. It generates additional hormones, such as human placental lactogen (hPL), which helps control the mother's metabolism and glucose levels, guaranteeing a consistent flow of nutrients to the growing child.

Overall, the placenta performs a key function in sustaining the embryonic stage of fetal development. It works as a lifeline, delivering oxygen, nutrition, and hormonal support to the growing embryo/fetus while aiding the evacuation of waste materials. The placenta's multifunctional skills are vital for the proper growth and development of the fetus during pregnancy.

The Fetal Stage

The fetal stage starts in the ninth week and continues until delivery. During this stage, the emphasis is on the development and refining of existing structures rather than the production of new organs.

The fetus continues fast development, and its dimensions start to mirror those of a full-term infant. Fingers and toes are completely developed, and the external genitalia begin to distinguish, however, it may be too early to confirm the baby's sex by ultrasound.

The fetal organs continue to grow and become more functioning. The respiratory system develops further, with the lungs starting to create surfactant, a chemical that helps the air sacs expand and keeps them from collapsing. The digestive system develops, and the intestines start to travel into the belly from the umbilical cord, where they originated.

The skeletal system ossifies, and bones grow harder and more defined. Muscle tone improves, and the fetus begins to demonstrate spontaneous movements, although these may not be noticed by the mother until later in the trimester.

By the conclusion of the first trimester, the fetus is roughly three inches in length and weighs about half an ounce. While still tiny and vulnerable, the fetus has made tremendous progress in terms of development and growth, laying the groundwork for continued maturity in the future trimesters.

Understanding the phases of fetal development during the first trimester gives an insight into the delicate process of producing new life. It is a monument to the extraordinary power of the human body to nurture and support the formation of a small, yet sophisticated, person.

Common Symptoms and Discomforts

The first trimester is generally accompanied by a variety of common symptoms and discomforts. While these experiences may differ from woman to woman, it is good to be informed of what you could expect:

- Morning Sickness

Morning sickness, marked by nausea and sometimes vomiting, is a typical symptom during the first trimester. Despite its name, it may occur at any hour of the day. To decrease morning sickness, consider eating small, frequent meals, avoiding spicy and oily foods, keeping hydrated, and getting enough rest.

- Fatigue

Feeling fatigued and drained is another frequent sensation in early pregnancy. Hormonal changes, increased blood production, and the need to raise a baby might contribute to this exhaustion. Make sure to prioritize relaxation, take short naps if required, and heed your body's cues to prevent overexertion.

- Breast Tenderness

As your body prepares for nursing, you may feel breast soreness and sensitivity. Wearing a supportive bra and administering warm compresses might help ease the pain.

- Frequent Urination

During pregnancy, your body generates more blood, and your kidneys work harder to clear waste. This increased blood flow and renal activity result in more frequent visits to the restroom. While it might be uncomfortable, keeping hydrated is vital for your general well-being and the proper growth of your kid.

Nutrition, Exercise, and Self-Care

Taking care of yourself throughout the first trimester is vital for your well-being and the well-being of your kid. Here are some recommendations and advice to maintain a healthy and balanced lifestyle

- Nutrition: Aim to have a nutritious and balanced diet that contains a range of fruits, vegetables, whole grains, lean proteins, and healthy fats. Pay attention to your body's changing dietary demands and consider integrating prenatal vitamins and supplements as prescribed by your healthcare professional.

- Exercise: Regular physical exercise during pregnancy may give several advantages, such as increasing mood, boosting energy levels, and encouraging healthy weight growth. However, it is crucial to talk with your healthcare physician before beginning or maintaining any fitness regimen. Low-impact exercises like walking, swimming, and prenatal yoga are typically safe and good alternatives.

- Self-Care: Pregnancy may be an emotionally and physically difficult period, so prioritizing self-care is vital. Engage in things that help you relax and decrease stress, like meditation, deep breathing exercises, prenatal massage, or pursuing hobbies you love. Adequate sleep, being hydrated, and having a good support system are other key components of self-care throughout pregnancy.

Possible Complications and Risks

While the first trimester is often a time of enthusiasm and expectation, it is crucial to be informed of various difficulties and hazards that may occur. These may include:

- Miscarriage: Miscarriage, the loss of a pregnancy before the 20th week, is sadly not uncommon and may occur for several causes, many of which are beyond your control. Signs of a probable miscarriage include vaginal bleeding, severe stomach discomfort, and cramping. If you encounter any of these symptoms, it is crucial to seek emergency medical assistance.

- Ectopic Pregnancy: An ectopic pregnancy develops when the fertilized egg implants outside the uterus, generally in the fallopian tube. It is a critical ailment that demands quick medical action, since it may create problems and represent a threat to the mother's health. Symptoms of an ectopic pregnancy may include stomach discomfort, vaginal bleeding, and shoulder ache. Prompt medical assessment is vital if you suspect an ectopic pregnancy.

Activities and Resources to Prepare for the Baby

The first trimester is an opportune time to start planning for the birth of your baby. Consider participating in the following activities and using available resources to facilitate a seamless transition into parenthood:

Prenatal Classes & Workshops

Attending prenatal seminars and workshops may equip you with vital knowledge and skills to manage pregnancy, delivery, and early parenting. These seminars frequently address subjects such as birthing education, breastfeeding, infant care, and postpartum support. Check with local hospitals, birthing centres, or community groups for available choices.

Creating a Birth Plan

A birth plan summarizes your preferences and wishes for the labour and delivery process. It might contain things like pain treatment alternatives, people you want there during delivery, and any particular requests or considerations. Discuss your birth plan with your healthcare practitioner and confirm that it corresponds with the regulations and practices of your selected birthing facility.

Setting Up the Nursery

Designing and setting up the baby's nursery may be a joyful and exciting undertaking. Consider establishing a peaceful and practical area that fulfills your baby's requirements. Research safe sleeping habits, pick suitable furniture and bedding, and arrange vital things including baby diapers, clothes, and feeding equipment.

Seeking Support

Building a support network is vital throughout pregnancy, and the first trimester is an appropriate time to start reaching out for help. Connect with other pregnant parents via online forums, support groups, or social media platforms. Engaging with experienced parents may give vital insights, guidance, and emotional support.

The first trimester represents the beginning of your remarkable adventure through pregnancy. From the physical and emotional changes you experience to the awe-inspiring phases of fetal development, this time provides the basis for your baby's growth. While the first trimester may bring along some discomforts and hazards, taking care of your physical and mental well-being, finding support, and participating in activities to prepare for your baby's birth will help assure a joyful and healthy experience. Remember to consult with your healthcare practitioner throughout your pregnancy experience, as they will guide and support you every step of the way.

Chapter 2

THE SECOND TRIMESTER

The second trimester of pregnancy is commonly referred to as the ***"honeymoon phase"*** since many women have a heightened sense of vitality and well-being during this time. It runs from week 13 to week 28 and is marked by major physical and emotional changes. In this chapter, we will delve into the various aspects of the second trimester, including the stages of fetal development and growth, physical and emotional changes, common symptoms and discomforts, nutrition and exercise, the risk of preterm labour, preparing for the baby, and important considerations such as prenatal testing, gender reveal, and baby registry.

Physical and Emotional Changes

During the second trimester, the pregnant body experiences dramatic modifications as the baby grows and develops. The uterus swells and rises over the pelvic area, becoming more apparent and giving the abdomen a rounder look. This expansion may lead to apparent changes in the woman's physique, such as a larger bust and a more distinct baby bump.

Another important physical change is the development of fetal movements, often known as *quickening.* As the baby gets more active, moms might feel light flutters or even forceful kicks and punches, building a feeling of connection and expectation.

In addition to physical changes, the second trimester brings about a spectrum of emotional adjustments. Many women find a heightened sense of confidence and excitement as they begin to embrace their pregnancy and connect with their developing baby. This stage is frequently accompanied by greater sensations of excitement and anticipation as the baby's movements grow more evident.

However, it is crucial to note that emotional changes might differ from person to person. Some women may also suffer mood changes, heightened emotions, or spells of worry. It is vital to seek help from loved ones and healthcare experts if these feelings become overpowering or interfere with normal functioning.

Stages of Fetal Development and Growth

Growth Spurt

The second trimester is a period of significant growth and development for the fetus. By the end of the fourth month, all the main organs and body systems have developed, and the baby's sex can frequently be verified by ultrasound. The baby's skin is covered with a thin covering of hair called lanugo, and eyebrows and eyelashes start to develop. The baby's senses, including hearing and taste, begin to develop, enabling them to react to external stimuli.

The Viability Milestone

Around the halfway point of the second trimester, often around week 24, the baby accomplishes a key milestone known as *viability.* Viability refers to the moment at which the infant has a possibility of surviving outside the womb with medical treatment. While the odds of survival at this point are still extremely low, medical improvements have raised the possibility of survival for kids delivered prematurely.

Fetal Movement and Sensory Development

During the second trimester, the baby's movements grow more obvious and synchronized. The mother may feel distinct kicks, rolls, and hiccups, which serve as a comforting indicator of the baby's well-being. The fetus also starts to develop its sense of touch, and studies show it may react to external stimuli, such as light and sound.

Common Symptoms and Discomforts

Morning Sickness Improvement

One of the nice developments in the second trimester is a decrease in morning sickness symptoms. Many women find relief from the nausea and vomiting that typically accompany early pregnancy. This enhancement permits individuals to restore their appetite and enjoy a larger range of meals.

Increased Energy Levels

With morning sickness fading, women generally enjoy a spike in energy throughout the second trimester. This increased vigour may be leveraged to participate in physical exercise, prepare for the baby's birth, or just enjoy the pregnancy adventure.

Round Ligament Pain

As the uterus grows, some women may have round ligament discomfort, characterized by acute or cramp-like feelings in the lower abdomen or groin. This pain is caused by the straining of the ligaments that support the uterus. Gentle stretching exercises, shifting position carefully, and utilizing supporting clothes will help ease this pain.

Braxton Hicks Contractions

Braxton Hicks contractions, often known as *practice contractions*, become more visible for many women during the second trimester. These irregular contractions prepare the uterus for labour but are often painless and do not signify the commencement of actual labour. Staying hydrated and shifting postures might help reduce any pain related to Braxton Hicks contractions.

Nutrition, Exercise, and Self-Care

Balanced Nutrition

Proper nutrition is vital throughout pregnancy, and the second trimester is no exception. A well-balanced diet rich in fruits, vegetables, whole grains, lean proteins, and healthy fats supplies the required nutrition for both the mother and the growing infant. Iron, calcium, folate, and omega-3 fatty acids are especially vital at this time. It is essential to speak with a healthcare physician or a trained dietitian to establish an adequate and tailored dietary plan.

Exercise and Physical Activity

Engaging in regular exercise throughout the second trimester may have various advantages. It helps to maintain general strength and flexibility, supports healthy weight gain, decreases the risk of gestational diabetes and pregnancy-related problems, and increases mood and energy levels. Low-impact exercises including walking, swimming, prenatal yoga, and stationary riding are typically safe and suggested. However, it is vital to contact a healthcare physician before beginning or adjusting any exercise plan.

Self-care and Emotional Well-being

Taking care of one's mental well-being is equally crucial throughout pregnancy. Engaging in activities that promote relaxation and stress reduction, such as mindfulness meditation, prenatal massages, and hobbies, might be useful. Seeking assistance from loved ones and attending pregnancy support groups or workshops may help give a feeling of community and emotional support. It is crucial to emphasize self-care and heed to one's body's demands.

Complications and Risks of Preterm Labor

Preterm labour, defined as the ***commencement of labour*** before 37 weeks of gestation, is a worry during the second trimester. It may lead to possible issues and challenges for both the newborn and the mother. Some risk factors for preterm labour include a history of preterm delivery, certain medical disorders, numerous pregnancies, and certain lifestyle variables. Pregnant persons must be aware of the signs and symptoms of preterm labour, such as frequent contractions, lower back discomfort, pelvic pressure, and vaginal bleeding, and seek urgent medical assistance if any of these symptoms arise.

Activities and Resources to Prepare for the Baby

The second trimester is an opportune time to start planning for the birth of the baby. Engaging in activities such as putting up the nursery, researching baby items, and attending childbirth education sessions may help parents feel more prepared and confident. It is also an appropriate moment to study resources, such as books, online forums, and parenting websites, that give vital information on many areas of infant care, nursing, and postpartum support.

Prenatal Testing, Gender Reveal, and Baby Registry

The second trimester generally involves critical prenatal tests to monitor the baby's health and screen for any possible abnormalities. These tests may include ultrasound scans, blood testing, Rh factor and antibody screening and genetic screenings. They give crucial information that may assist guide medical treatment and decision-making throughout the pregnancy.

- **Ultrasound:** Ultrasound imaging is a frequently used prenatal test that employs sound waves to provide pictures of the growing baby. During the second trimester, an anatomy ultrasound, also known as a level 2 ultrasound, is often conducted between weeks 18 and 22. This comprehensive ultrasound examination analyzes the baby's anatomy, including the brain, heart, spine, limbs, and internal organs. It may also reveal information on the baby's gender if desired. For many pregnant parents, finding out the baby's gender is a joyful time. The second trimester is generally when a baby's gender may be established by ultrasound if desired. Some parents may opt to host a gender reveal event to commemorate this milestone with relatives and friends.

Additionally, ultrasound measures of the baby's growth and amniotic fluid level, may be conducted to monitor development.

- **Multiple Marker Screening:**

Multiple marker screening, often known as the quad screen or the triple screen, is a blood test that tests for various genetic disorders and chromosomal abnormalities in the foetus. It examines the levels of different chemicals in the mother's blood, including alpha-fetoprotein (AFP), human chorionic gonadotropin (hCG), estriol, and inhibin A. The data, coupled with maternal age and gestational age, are used to determine the risk of disorders such as Down syndrome, trisomy 18, and neural tube abnormalities. If the findings show an elevated risk, additional diagnostic testing may be required.

- **Glucose Challenge Test:** The glucose challenge test (GCT) is a screening test for gestational diabetes, a kind of diabetes that may arise during pregnancy. It is commonly conducted between weeks 24 and 28 of pregnancy. The test comprises drinking a sweet beverage containing a specified quantity of glucose, followed by a blood test to assess the blood sugar level. Elevated blood sugar levels may signal the need for additional testing, such as the glucose tolerance test, to confirm gestational diabetes.

- **Rh Factor and Antibody Screening:** Rh factor and antibody screening is a blood test that identifies whether a woman is Rh positive or Rh negative. Rh factor refers to a particular protein located on the surface of red blood cells. If a woman is Rh negative and her baby is Rh positive, there is a danger of Rh incompatibility, where the mother's immune system may release antibodies that might destroy the baby's red blood cells. This test helps identify Rh-negative women who may need extra monitoring and treatment during pregnancy.

Rh incompatibility during pregnancy might offer some dangers to the infant. Here are some of the possible issues linked with Rh incompatibility:

1. Hemolytic illness of the Newborn (HDN): Rh incompatibility may lead to hemolytic illness of the newborn, often known as Rh disease. If a Rh-negative mother is sensitized to the Rh factor (by exposure to Rh-positive blood, generally during a prior pregnancy or blood transfusion), her immune system may create antibodies termed Rh antibodies. These antibodies may penetrate the placenta and assault the red blood cells of a Rh-positive infant. This may result in the breakdown of red blood cells and lead to anaemia and other issues in the infant.

2. Jaundice: As a consequence of the breakdown of red blood cells, the newborn may develop a disease called jaundice. Jaundice develops when there is an excess of bilirubin, a yellow pigment generated

during the breakdown of red blood cells. Elevated levels of bilirubin may cause yellowing of the skin and eyes and may need treatment to avoid more serious problems.

3. Anaemia: The breakdown of red blood cells may lead to anaemia in the infant. Anaemia is a disorder defined by a reduction in the number of red blood cells or a low quantity of haemoglobin, which is responsible for transporting oxygen in the blood. Severe anaemia may damage the baby's growth and development and may need medical intervention.

4. Hydrops Fetalis: In rare situations of severe Rh incompatibility, a disorder termed hydrops fetalis may arise. Hydrops fetalis is defined by abnormal fluid collection in two or more fetal compartments, such as the belly, chest, or skin. It may result in

severe oedema, respiratory discomfort, and heart failure in the newborn, and it may be life-threatening.

To avoid Rh incompatibility issues, Rh-negative women who are at risk of sensitization (such as those who have not been sensitized previously) are routinely administered Rh immunoglobulin (RhIG) during pregnancy. RhIG is an injection that may prevent the mother from developing Rh antibodies. It is normally provided during the 28th week of pregnancy and within 72 hours after birth if the infant is Rh-positive. RhIG may help safeguard future pregnancies from Rh incompatibility issues.

Rh-negative women must have adequate prenatal care and follow the recommendations of their healthcare professionals to reduce the dangers associated with Rh incompatibility.

- **Group B Streptococcus (GBS) Screening:** Group B Streptococcus is a kind of bacterium that may be found in the vagina or rectum of certain pregnant women. GBS screening is commonly conducted between weeks 35 and 37 of pregnancy. A swab is collected from the vagina and rectum to test for the presence of GBS. If GBS is found, the mother may get antibiotics during birth to lessen the risk of spreading the illness to the baby.

It is crucial to remember that these tests are optional and their usage may vary based on the healthcare professional and the individual conditions of the pregnancy. It is suggested to review the various prenatal tests with a healthcare practitioner to establish whether tests are suitable and essential for each particular pregnancy.

Baby Registry

Creating a baby registry is a sensible approach to preparing for the baby's arrival and ensuring that vital products are accessible. Many companies offer registry services, enabling parents to construct a list of baby basics, such as clothes, diapers, furnishings, and feeding gear. Family and friends may then go to the registry while purchasing presents for the expecting parents

The second trimester is a transforming and joyful period in pregnancy. It is marked by bodily changes, emotional alterations, and considerable fetal growth. While typical symptoms and discomforts may emerge, adequate self-care, diet, and exercise may help promote well-being. Understanding the risks of preterm labour and obtaining adequate prenatal care is critical. Engaging in activities to prepare for the baby and exploring alternatives such as prenatal testing, gender reveal, and baby registry may further enrich the pregnancy experience.

Chapter 3

THE THIRD TRIMESTER

The third trimester of pregnancy, which covers from week 28 to the delivery of the baby, is a pivotal phase fraught with substantial physical and mental changes. During this period, the baby undergoes fast growth, while the pregnant mother experiences the last phases of pregnancy. In this chapter, we will explore the various aspects of the third trimester, including the physical and emotional changes, stages of fetal development, common symptoms and discomforts, nutrition and exercise recommendations, self-care tips, potential complications, and preparations for the baby's arrival.

Physical and Emotional Changes

As the third-trimester advances, the pregnant mother may experience a variety of physical and emotional changes. Physically, the belly continues to develop as the baby acquires weight and prepares for delivery. This may lead to increased pain, backaches, and shortness of breath as the enlarging uterus exerts pressure on the diaphragm and other organs. The mother may also feel frequent urination, swelling in the hands and feet, and difficulties sleeping owing to pain.

Emotionally, the third trimester may offer a combination of enthusiasm, expectation, and worry. The anticipated birth of the baby may lead to heightened emotions, mood swings, and nesting tendencies. It is usual for expecting parents to experience a variety of emotions, from excitement and delight to concern and dread about childbirth, parenting, and the baby's well-being. The mother must take time for self-care, seek support from loved ones, and talk freely about her emotions.

Stages of Fetal Development and Growth

During the third trimester, the baby experiences amazing growth and development. In the early part of this trimester, the baby's organs continue to progress, and the brain develops fast. The lungs also undergo essential adaptations to prepare for breathing outside the womb. The baby's movements may become more obvious and frequent when room in the uterus becomes restricted.

As the due date approaches, the baby may relax into a head-down position in preparation for delivery. The baby's senses, like as hearing and vision, continue to develop, and they may even react to external stimuli, such as noises and light. Towards the conclusion of the third trimester, the baby's weight increase accelerates, and the body stores more fat to offer insulation and energy reserves for the newborn period.

Common Symptoms and Discomforts of Late Pregnancy

The third trimester is commonly linked with a variety of common symptoms and discomforts. These include:

1. **Braxton Hicks Contractions:** These are small, irregular contractions that may be felt while the uterus prepares for childbirth. They may be

recognised from genuine labour contractions since they are typically painless and do not rise in strength or frequency.

2. **Heartburn. and Indigestion:** The developing uterus may press on the stomach, resulting in digestive difficulties including heartburn and indigestion. Eating smaller, more frequent meals and avoiding hot or oily foods will help reduce these symptoms.

3. **Swelling and Fluid Retention:** Many women suffer swelling, especially in the hands, feet, and ankles, during late pregnancy. This is related to fluid retention and increased pressure on the blood vessels. Elevating the feet and wearing comfortable, supportive shoes may assist in minimising oedema.

4. **Shortness of Breath:** As the uterus swells, it may press on the diaphragm and restrict lung capacity, leading to symptoms of breathlessness. Taking regular rests, keeping excellent posture, and doing deep breathing exercises might help control this condition.

5. **Weariness:** The physical demands of pregnancy, along with hormonal changes and trouble sleeping, might lead to greater weariness throughout the third trimester. It is crucial to prioritize rest, develop a regular sleep regimen, and seek assistance when required.

Nutrition, Exercise, and Self-Care

Maintaining a healthy lifestyle throughout the third trimester is vital for the well-being of both the mother and the baby. Proper diet, frequent exercise, and self-care habits may promote a healthy pregnancy. Here are some tips:

1. Nutrition: Focus on a balanced diet that includes a range of fruits, vegetables, whole grains, lean meats, and healthy fats. Ensure an appropriate diet of vitamins and minerals, especially iron, calcium, and folic acid. Stay hydrated by drinking lots of water and avoid the use of coffee, processed meals, and sugary snacks.

2. Exercise: Engage in frequent, low-impact workouts like walking, swimming, prenatal yoga, or prenatal aerobics. These exercises may help maintain fitness, enhance circulation, minimize pain, and prepare the body for birth. Consult with a healthcare physician before beginning or adjusting an exercise plan.

3. Self-Care: Take time for self-care activities that promote relaxation and emotional well-being. This may involve techniques like meditation, deep breathing exercises, prenatal massage, warm baths, and listening to relaxing music. Engage in things that offer delight and help release stress as reading, spending time in nature, or pursuing hobbies.

4. Rest and Sleep: Get adequate rest and prioritize sleep to manage tiredness. Create a pleasant sleep

environment, set a nighttime ritual, and utilise pillows or other supports to reach a comfortable posture for sleep.

Possible Complications and Risks

While most pregnancies develop normally, it is vital to be aware of possible issues that might occur during the third trimester. Three frequent problems are preeclampsia, gestational diabetes, and placenta previa.

Preeclampsia: Preeclampsia is a disorder characterized by high blood pressure and damage to organs, such as the liver and kidneys, during pregnancy. It may lead to difficulties for both the mother and the baby if left untreated. Symptoms may include high blood pressure, oedema, unexpected weight gain, and changes in eyesight. Regular prenatal check-ups and monitoring of blood pressure and urine may help diagnose preeclampsia early.

Managing and avoiding preeclampsia during the third trimester is of the highest significance for the health and well-being of both the mother and the baby. Preeclampsia is a disorder characterized by high blood pressure and damage to organs, such as the liver and kidneys, during pregnancy. Here are several methods that might aid in controlling and avoiding preeclampsia:

- Regular Prenatal Care: Attending all regular prenatal sessions is critical for early diagnosis and treatment of preeclampsia. Healthcare personnel will monitor blood pressure, urine protein levels, and other pertinent measures to detect any symptoms of preeclampsia. They may also prescribe further testing, such as blood tests and ultrasounds, to examine the health of both the mother and the baby.

- Blood Pressure Monitoring: Regular monitoring of blood pressure is vital in controlling preeclampsia. If high blood pressure is diagnosed, healthcare experts may offer lifestyle adjustments, medicines, or other treatments to reduce blood pressure and avoid additional issues.

- Healthy Diet: Following a well-balanced diet rich in fruits, vegetables, whole grains, lean meats, and healthy fats is vital for general health and may aid in treating preeclampsia. Avoiding high salt consumption and processed meals might also be useful. It is essential to speak with a healthcare physician or a qualified dietitian for individualised dietary suggestions.

- Adequate Rest and Sleep: Sufficient rest and sleep are vital for controlling preeclampsia. Fatigue and stress might lead to higher blood pressure levels. It is crucial for expecting moms to prioritize rest, create a regular sleep regimen, and seek assistance from loved ones to avoid stress.

- Physical Activity: Engaging in frequent, low-impact activities, as directed by a healthcare expert, may aid in treating and avoiding preeclampsia. Physical exercise boosts circulation, decreases stress, and helps maintain general fitness. However, it is vital to talk with a healthcare physician before beginning or adjusting an exercise plan during pregnancy.

- Medication and Supplements: In certain circumstances, healthcare practitioners may recommend drugs to treat high blood pressure linked with preeclampsia. Additionally, physicians may offer supplements like as calcium and low-dose aspirin to lower the risk of preeclampsia. It is crucial to follow healthcare experts' instructions about drug and supplement usage.

- Monitoring Symptoms: Expectant moms should be aware of the symptoms of preeclampsia, which may include high blood pressure, oedema, abrupt weight gain, changes in eyesight, severe headaches, and upper abdomen discomfort. Promptly reporting any concerned symptoms to a healthcare physician is critical for early discovery and effective therapy.

- Stress Reduction: Managing stress is vital for general well-being and may aid in avoiding preeclampsia. Engaging in relaxation methods like as deep breathing exercises, meditation, prenatal yoga, or getting help from a therapist or support groups might be therapeutic.

It is crucial to remember that although these steps may aid in controlling and avoiding preeclampsia, they may not guarantee total avoidance or a cure. Close monitoring by healthcare practitioners and following their suggestions are vital for the treatment of preeclampsia.

Gestational Diabetes: Gestational diabetes is a kind of diabetes that develops during pregnancy. It is characterized by elevated blood sugar levels that might offer dangers to both the mother and the fetus. Regular blood sugar monitoring, a balanced diet, exercise, and, in some circumstances, medication or insulin treatment may help control gestational diabetes.

Placenta Previa: Placenta previa occurs when the placenta partly or fully covers the cervix, leading to possible problems during labour and delivery. Among the signs and symptoms include third trimester virginal bleeding. Close monitoring by a healthcare practitioner and probable revisions to the birth plan may be required.

Pregnant moms need to attend all planned prenatal checkups, report any concerns or symptoms to healthcare professionals, and follow their recommendations for monitoring and treatment of these issues.

Activities and Resources to Prepare for the Baby

The third trimester is an opportune time to prepare for the birth of the baby. Here are some activities and resources that might help:

1. **Childbirth Education programmes:** Consider enrolling in childbirth education programmes, which include knowledge of labour, delivery, and infant care. These seminars may help pregnant parents feel more prepared and confident.

2. **Baby Registry and Shopping:** Create a baby registry to assist arrange the required products for the baby. Research and make educated decisions regarding products including baby cribs, car seats,

strollers, and nursing gear. Consider buying basics in advance to reduce last-minute stress.

3. **Preparing the Nursery:** Set up the nursery, including furniture, bedding, and decorations. Make sure the area is secure by baby proofing electrical outlets and securing furniture to avoid mishaps.

4. **Packing the Hospital Bag:** As the due date approaches, prepare a hospital bag with necessities for labour, delivery, and the postpartum period. This may contain comfortable attire, toiletries, necessary paperwork, food, and things for the baby.

Labor Signs, Birth Plan, and Hospital Bag

Towards the conclusion of the third trimester, it is crucial to be acquainted with labour signals, establish a birth plan, and have a packed hospital bag. Familiarize yourself with indicators of labour, including regular contractions, rupture of membranes (water breaking), and bloody shows. Discuss your birth preferences with your healthcare practitioner and prepare a birth plan that describes your choices for pain treatment, labour positions, and other elements of delivery. Pack a hospital bag with important goods for yourself, your spouse, and the baby, including vital paperwork, comfortable clothes, toiletries, and items for the infant.

Exercises that might Help Labour

Engaging in regular exercise throughout pregnancy, even the third trimester, may have several advantages, including preparing the body for labour and delivery. However, it's vital to contact your healthcare professional before beginning or adjusting an exercise regimen, as they may give individualized advice based on your unique health and pregnancy.

Here are some usually advised workouts throughout the third trimester that may assist prepare for labour:

1. **Walking:** Walking is a low-impact activity that may be readily included in your everyday routine. It

helps to increase cardiovascular fitness, maintain muscular tone, and stimulate circulation. Walking also stimulates the baby to descend into the pelvis, which may assist in the course of labour.

2. **Prenatal Yoga:** Prenatal yoga is a mild kind of exercise that focuses on stretching, relaxation, and breathing techniques. It may assist enhance flexibility, strengthen the muscles required for labour, and promote relaxation and stress reduction. Look for prenatal yoga courses particularly developed for pregnant ladies.

3. **Pelvic Floor Exercises:** The pelvic floor muscles serve a crucial function in maintaining the uterus and pelvic organs, as well as during labour and delivery. Exercises like Kegels may assist in strengthening these muscles, which may increase

their capacity to support the baby and aid the pushing phase of labour.

4. **Squats:** Squats are a useful workout for opening up the pelvis and strengthening the lower body muscles. They may assist, promote flexibility and prepare the body for the birthing position. It is vital to practice squats with good technique and assistance, such as utilizing a stability ball or holding onto a firm item for balance.

5. **Prenatal Pilates:** Prenatal Pilates focuses on strengthening the core muscles, improving posture, and developing body awareness. It may assist in maintaining muscular tone, stability, and flexibility, which are essential throughout pregnancy and birth. Look for prenatal Pilates sessions offered by

qualified instructors who are experienced in dealing with pregnant ladies.

6. **Swimming:** Swimming and water aerobics give a low-impact activity that helps reduce the pressure on joints and ligaments. The buoyancy of water supports the body, making it simpler to move and exercise. Swimming may also help decrease swelling and pain associated with pregnancy.

Remember to listen to your body and alter workouts as required. Avoid activities that place excessive pressure on your joints or entail a high risk of falling or abdominal damage. Stay hydrated, wear comfortable clothes and supportive footwear, and take breaks as required.

Always check with your healthcare practitioner before beginning or maintaining any workout regimen during pregnancy. They can give advice depending on your unique health situation and any possible dangers or contraindications.

How to Execute the KEGEL Workout

Kegel exercises, commonly known as pelvic floor exercises, are meant to strengthen the muscles of the pelvic floor. These exercises may be advantageous throughout pregnancy, as they assist support the weight of the developing uterus, enhance bladder control, and can aid in the pushing phase of delivery. Here's a step-by-step tutorial on how to execute Kegel exercises correctly:

1. **Identify the Pelvic Floor Muscles:**

Before you can start practicing Kegel exercises, it's vital to identify the right muscles. The best method to achieve this is to envision halting the flow of pee midway. The muscles that you activate to achieve this are called the pelvic floor muscles.

2. **Find a Comfortable Position:** You may practice Kegel exercises in numerous postures, such as sitting, lying down, or standing. Choose a posture that is comfortable for you and enables you to concentrate on the activity.

3. **Contract the Pelvic Floor Muscles:**

Once you have recognised the pelvic floor muscles, contract them by squeezing and pulling them upward. Imagine drawing them in and elevating them as if you are attempting to hold in pee or gas. Be cautious not to contract the muscles in your belly, buttocks, or thighs. The attention should be on the pelvic floor.

4. **Hold the Contraction**: Once you have clenched the pelvic floor muscles, hold the contraction for a few seconds. Start with holding for 3-5 seconds and then increase the time as you gain stronger. Remember to breathe normally throughout the hold and avoid tensing other portions of your body.

5. **Release and Relax**: After holding the contraction, release the pelvic floor muscles and

allow them to relax totally. Rest for a few seconds before commencing the following repeat.

6. **Repeat the Exercise:** Aim to execute 10-20 repetitions of Kegel exercises in a row. If you're a newbie, you may need to start with fewer repetitions and gradually build up. As you get more comfortable and experienced, you may increase the amount of sets throughout the day.

7. **Do frequently:** To notice the advantages of Kegel exercises, it's vital to do them frequently. Aim for at least three sets of workouts each day. You may include them in your everyday schedule, such as performing a set in the morning, afternoon, and evening.

Remember, it's crucial to practice Kegel exercises properly to achieve the best effect. Avoid squeezing other muscles, such as the buttocks or thighs, and concentrate entirely on the pelvic floor muscles. If you're unclear if you're completing Kegels properly or have any concerns, it's always a good idea to contact your healthcare physician or a pelvic floor physical therapist who can give assistance and tailored suggestions.

Note: Kegel exercises are typically safe for most pregnant women, but it's always a good idea to contact your healthcare professional before beginning any workout regimen during pregnancy, particularly, if you are concerned about any underlying medical conditions.

Precautions for the KEGEL Workout

While Kegel exercises are typically safe and useful for most individuals, even during pregnancy, it's crucial to keep a few considerations in mind to ensure you're completing them properly and safely. Here are some measures to consider:

- Consult with your healthcare provider: Before starting or continuing with any exercise routine, including Kegel exercises, it's best to consult with your healthcare provider, especially if you have any underlying medical conditions, such as pelvic pain, urinary incontinence, or a history of pelvic floor dysfunction. They may give individualized coaching and guarantee that Kegel exercises are appropriate for you.

- Identify the right muscles: Take the time to correctly identify and isolate the pelvic floor muscles before conducting Kegel exercises. This will assist kíin guaranteeing that you're targeting the proper muscles and not mistakenly activating other neighbouring muscles.

- Avoid overexertion: While it's vital to test and develop the pelvic floor muscles, it's as critical not to overexert them. Start with shorter contractions and progressively increase the time as your muscles grow stronger. Avoid straining or pushing too hard, since this might lead to muscular exhaustion or soreness.

- Breathe normally: Remember to breathe properly throughout Kegel exercises. Avoid holding your breath, since it may produce unneeded stress in the body. Inhale and exhale normally while you do the contractions and relaxations.

- Don't stop the urine flow: While it's encouraged to identify the pelvic floor muscles by momentarily halting the flow of urine, it's crucial not to utilise this as a regular practice for conducting Kegel exercises. Interrupting the urine flow repeatedly might disturb normal bladder function and may raise the risk of urinary tract infections.

- Be constant and patient: Like any activity, consistency is crucial. Aim to execute Kegel exercises frequently, preferably three times a day, to observe the effects over time. However, be patient with your development. It may take many weeks or even months to detect major changes in pelvic floor strength and bladder control.

- Seek professional assistance if needed: If you're unclear about completing Kegel exercises properly, feeling pain or discomfort, or if you're not seeing the desired results, consider obtaining guidance from a pelvic floor physical therapist. They may give specialized evaluation, coaching, and extra exercises or strategies to suit your unique requirements.

Keep in mind that every individual has a different body, so what suits one person may not suit another. It's vital to listen to your body, start cautiously, and alter the workouts as required. If you suffer any pain, discomfort, or strange symptoms while or after practicing Kegel exercises, it's suggested to quit and talk with your healthcare physician.

The third trimester of pregnancy is a period of major physical and emotional changes for both the mother and the baby. By recognising and planning for these changes, managing typical discomforts, and being aware of potential issues, expecting parents may traverse this time with confidence and secure the best possible results for themselves and their babies. Taking care of physical and mental well-being, seeking assistance, and participating in preparations may help to a smooth transition into the latter months of pregnancy and the birth of the new family member.

Chapter 4

LABOUR & DELIVERY

Labour and delivery are key milestones in the experience of pregnancy. In this chapter, we will explore the different types and stages of labour, discuss pain relief and induction options, delve into possible complications and interventions, provide tips for coping with labour, address the role of the partner and birth team, suggest activities and resources for preparation, and introduce the topics of newborn care, breastfeeding, and postpartum recovery.

Types and Stages of Labor

Early Labor

Early labour, also known as the ***latent phase***, is the early stage of labour. During this phase, the cervix progressively softens, thins out (effaces), and starts to dilate. Contractions may be irregular and moderate at first, frequently mimicking menstruation cramps. This period may linger for hours or even days, and it is usual for women to feel a variety of emotions at this time. It is advisable to remain at home during early labour, rest, and perform comfort measures such as relaxation methods, breathing exercises, and modest physical activity.

Active Labor

Active labour signals the shift to increasingly powerful and regular contractions. The cervix continues to dilate, often reaching approximately 4 to 7 cm. Contractions get stronger, longer, and closer together, generally happening every 3 to 5 minutes. During this stage, it is preferable to proceed to the birthing place, as labour is continuing, and medical personnel can monitor the mother and offer necessary assistance. Pain management measures, like breathing exercises, relaxation techniques, and position modifications, may assist deal with the growing severity of contractions.

Transition

Transition is the last step of the active stage of work. The cervix further dilates, reaching roughly 8 to 10 centimeters. Contractions are severe, lasting for roughly 60 to 90 seconds and happening every 2 to 3 minutes. Many women feel a variety of emotions at this time, including anger, restlessness, and self-doubt. It is vital to stay focused and employ pain management measures, including breathing exercises, relaxation, and ongoing support from the delivery team.

Second Stage: Pushing and Delivery

The second stage of labour occurs when the cervix is completely dilated. It involves the vigorous pushing and delivery of the baby. Women frequently have a strong need to push at this stage, and the baby's head starts to descend into the delivery canal. With direction from the healthcare practitioner, the woman pushes during contractions to help guide the baby through the delivery canal. This stage might range from a few minutes to a few hours. It is crucial to preserve energy between contractions and follow the instructions of the healthcare expert about pushing tactics and postures.

Third Stage: Delivery of the Placenta

After the baby is delivered, the third stage of labour includes the delivery of the placenta. The uterus continues to contract, forcing the placenta to detach from the uterine wall. The healthcare practitioner will examine the mother's condition and instruct her on when to push or use controlled cord traction to deliver the placenta. This stage is generally shorter and less severe than the preceding phases.

Pain Relief and Induction Options

Pain Relief

Labour may be accompanied by tremendous pain, and numerous pain treatment alternatives are available to assist, manage discomfort. These alternatives include:

Non-Pharmacological Methods

Non-pharmacological pain treatment approaches attempt to deliver comfort and relaxation without the need for drugs. Some typical approaches include breathing exercises, relaxation techniques, massage, water immersion or bathing, posture modifications, hot or cold packs, and aromatherapy. These approaches may be beneficial in lowering discomfort and increasing a feeling of control during delivery.

Pharmacological Methods

Pharmacological pain management solutions entail the use of drugs to relieve pain during delivery. These alternatives include:

- Analgesics: Pain-relieving drugs, such as opioids, may be provided either an injection or intravenously to assist control the pain. They may help take the edge off the pain but may not eradicate it. These drugs may alter the mother's attentiveness and may have repercussions for the baby.

- Epidural Analgesia: Epidural anaesthesia is a regularly utilized therapy for pain reduction during delivery. It includes the delivery of local anaesthetics and occasionally opioids into the epidural area, numbing the lower half of the body. This approach gives good pain relief, enabling the mother to relax and save energy. However, it may have negative effects such as low blood pressure and the requirement for assisted delivery.

Induction of Labour

In certain instances, labour may need to be induced, meaning it begins artificially before it begins naturally. Reasons for labour induction might include post-term pregnancy, medical issues, fetal distress, or other maternal or fetal reasons. procedures of labour induction may include the use of synthetic hormones such as oxytocin or prostaglandins to trigger contractions, rupturing the amniotic membranes, or mechanical procedures like cervical ripening with a balloon catheter. Induction of labour should be undertaken under the advice of healthcare experts, and the risks and benefits should be carefully addressed.

Complications and Interventions during Labor and Delivery

Complications during Labor

Labor and delivery may occasionally entail problems that necessitate medical treatment. Some of such difficulties include:

Protracted Labor: When labour advances slowly, it is termed protracted labour. This may be attributed to several circumstances, such as inadequate contractions, a huge baby, or a limited pelvis. Medical procedures, such as augmentation with synthetic hormones or aided delivery with devices like forceps or suction, may be essential.

Fetal Distress:

Fetal distress refers to symptoms that the baby is not enduring labour well. This might be suggested by aberrant heart rate patterns or diminished fetal movement. It may need quick steps, such as altering the mother's position, providing oxygen, or conducting an emergency cesarean section.

Umbilical cord issues:

Sometimes, the umbilical cord may become squeezed or prolapsed, leading to possible issues for the newborn. Prompt treatment, such as altering the mother's position or conducting an emergency cesarean section, may be essential to release the strain on the chord and guarantee the baby's well-being.

Interventions during Delivery

During the delivery process, healthcare personnel may need to utilize interventions to guarantee the safety of both the mother and the infant. Some typical interventions include:

Episiotomy: An episiotomy is a surgical incision done in the perineum (the region between the vagina and anus) to expand the vaginal opening during birth. While this operation was originally regular, it is now conducted selectively depending on the unique conditions. Episiotomies may be essential if the infant has to be delivered rapidly or if there is worry about serious tearing.

Instrumental Delivery: Instrumental delivery includes the use of devices, such as forceps or vacuum extractors, to help in the birth of the baby. These tools are gently put on the baby's head to guide and help in the birth process. Instrumental delivery is normally reserved for circumstances when there is a need to hasten birth or aid with particular challenges.

Cesarean Section: A cesarean section, sometimes referred to as a C-section, is a medical operation in which the baby is delivered via an incision in the mother's belly and uterus. It may be scheduled in advance or done as an emergency operation if there are difficulties that make vaginal delivery hazardous or if labour is not progressing as predicted.

Coping with Labor and Delivery

Personalized Coping Strategies

Every woman's experience of labour and delivery is unique, and coping tactics may differ. Here are some common strategies to assist deal with labour

- Education and Preparedness: Attend childbirth education courses to learn about the labour process, pain management strategies, and relaxation methods. Understanding what to anticipate may help ease anxiety and allow you to make educated choices throughout childbirth.

- Supportive Environment: Surround yourself with a supportive delivery team, which may include your spouse, family members, or a doula. Their presence, encouragement, and advocacy may give emotional and physical support throughout the procedure.

- Breathing and Relaxation methods: Practice deep breathing, visualization, and relaxation methods to help manage pain and decrease stress. These practices may foster a feeling of calm and help you remain focused throughout contractions.

- Position Changes: Experiment with various postures, like walking, sitting on a birth ball, or using a rocking rocker, to determine what is most comfortable for you. Changing postures may assist reduce pressure, support appropriate fetal placement, and increase labour progress.

- Hydrotherapy: Consider employing water immersion, such as having a warm shower or labouring in a birthing pool, since water may give pain relief and relaxation.

- Ongoing Assistance: Having ongoing assistance from a trusted companion, such as a spouse or doula, may improve the delivery experience. Their presence and encouragement may bring confidence and help you feel supported during labour.

Pain Management Techniques

In addition to customized coping tactics, many pain management approaches might be beneficial during labour:

- Breathing Techniques: Practice calm, deep breathing during contractions. Focus on breathing deeply through your nose and expelling gently through your mouth. This might help you relax and manage discomfort.
- Massage and Counterpressure: Gentle massage or applying pressure to particular

regions, such as the lower back or hips, might assist ease pain during labour. Experiment with various ways and discover what works best for you.

- Heat and Cold Therapy: Applying heat or cold might give relief during childbirth. Use warm compresses, take a warm shower for relaxation, or apply cold packs to areas of pain.

- TENS (Transcutaneous Electrical Nerve Stimulation): TENS is a treatment that employs a tiny portable device that delivers low-voltage electrical currents to particular parts of the body via electrodes put on the skin.

Chapter 5

THE FOURTH TRIMESTER

The fourth trimester refers to the time after delivery **(*postpartum*)**, often lasting approximately six weeks, during which parents endure substantial physical and emotional changes as they adjust to caring for a baby. It is a key moment of adjustment and learning. Let's discuss the many characteristics of the fourth trimester in depth.

Physical and Emotional Changes in the Postpartum Period

During the postpartum period, the body goes through numerous essential changes as it heals after delivery. One of the important processes is uterine involution, which is the shrinkage of the uterus back to its pre-pregnancy size and location. This procedure includes the tightening of uterine muscles to evacuate extra blood and tissue left during pregnancy.

Hormonal levels also experience major alterations during this period. Estrogen and progesterone, the hormones that were elevated throughout pregnancy, diminish significantly after delivery. These hormonal fluctuations might contribute to mood swings, exhaustion, and night sweats. It is crucial to know that these changes are natural and transient.

Additionally, the body undergoes a mending process for perineal tissues, whether after a vaginal delivery or a cesarean section. The perineum may incur tears or episiotomies after vaginal delivery, which need adequate care and attention for healing. For people who have had a cesarean section, the incision site needs particular care to avoid infection and promote recovery.

Breast alterations are also frequent during the postpartum period. Engorgement, a condition in which the breasts grow large and painful as they swell with milk, is typical. Proper latch and placement while breastfeeding are vital to guarantee adequate milk transfer and reduce pain. As breastfeeding continues, the breasts will respond to the baby's eating habits and milk supply will be adjusted according to demand.

Emotionally, the postpartum period may be a rollercoaster of emotions for new parents. Feelings of excitement, tiredness, mood swings, and worry are all-natural. Hormonal fluctuations, sleep loss, and the adjustment to the new role of motherhood might contribute to these emotional shifts. Parents must acknowledge and normalize these sentiments and seek help from healthcare experts, family, and friends.

Caring for a Newborn

Caring for a baby entails different things that demand care and awareness. Let's study the key components of infant care, including feeding, diapering, washing, sleep patterns, and calming strategies.

Feeding an infant is a significant issue for parents. Breastfeeding is typically advised as the greatest way of sustenance for newborns owing to its multiple advantages. It offers necessary nutrition, and antibodies, and promotes bonding. Proper latch and placement are vital for effective breastfeeding, and getting support from lactation consultants and healthcare experts may be useful.

For parents who prefer to bottle feed, whether with expressed breast milk or formula, it is crucial to follow safe feeding techniques. This involves sanitizing bottles and nipples, preparing formula according to prescribed recommendations, and ensuring the infant is held in a comfortable and supported posture while feeding. Paying attention to the baby's hunger and fullness signs is also vital.

Diapering is a crucial element of infant care to keep the baby clean, dry, and comfortable. Having a supply of diapers, wipes, and diaper rash treatment is vital. Diapers should be changed often to avoid diaper rash and maintain adequate cleanliness.

Understanding a newborn's sleep habits is vital for their well-being and the parents' rest. Newborns sleep for varied lengths throughout the day and night, with intervals of awake for feeding and diaper changes. Following safe sleep habits such as laying the infant on their back to sleep, utilising a solid and level sleeping surface, and keeping the sleep environment free from risks is crucial.

Soothing practices may help soothe a newborn and bring comfort. Swaddling, which includes covering the infant tightly in a blanket, may imitate the experience of being in the womb and generate a sense of security. Gentle rocking or utilizing a baby swing or a rocking chair may also help calm a fussy infant. Additionally, utilizing white noise, such as a sound generator or calm music, may produce a peaceful atmosphere.

These are only some of the crucial parts of caring for a baby throughout the fourth trimester. Each infant is unique, and parents should follow their instincts while obtaining help from healthcare experts and experienced caregivers.

Postpartum Depression

Postpartum depression is a mental illness that affects some parents after delivery. It is characterized by emotions of melancholy, worry, and weariness that are more acute and persistent than the "baby blues" that many new parents experience. Postpartum depression may make it tough to completely participate in everyday activities and care for the infant. Let's investigate this ailment in greater depth, including its indicators, causes, and treatment techniques.

Signs of Postpartum Depression

Postpartum depression may show in numerous ways, and the signs and symptoms may vary from person to person. Some typical indicators of postpartum depression include:

- Persistent emotions of melancholy, despair, or emptiness.
- Loss of interest or pleasure in activities that were formerly pleasant.
- Fatigue and lack of energy, even with proper rest.
- Changes in appetite, either a major rise or reduction.
- Difficulty sleeping or sleeping excessively.

- Irritability, restlessness, or agitation.

- Feelings of guilt, worthlessness, or excessive self-blame.

- Trouble focusing, making judgements, or remembering facts.

- Thoughts of hurting oneself or, in severe cases, the baby.

Causes of Postpartum Depression

Postpartum depression is thought to be caused by a combination of environmental, emotional physiological factors while the precise causes are not fully understood. Some probable reasons include

1. Hormonal changes: After delivery, there is a significant reduction in hormones like estrogen and progesterone, which may lead to mood swings and mental instability.

2. History of mental health issues: Individuals having a personal or family history of depression, anxiety, or other mental health problems may have an increased chance of developing postpartum depression.

3. Stress and life changes: The responsibilities and difficulties of caring for a baby, along with sleep loss and lifestyle alterations, may raise stress levels and contribute to depression.

4. Lack of social support: Limited support from partners, family, or friends may aggravate feelings of isolation and make it more tough to manage postpartum issues.

5. Previous traumatic experiences: A history of trauma, such as abuse or a terrible birthing experience, may raise the chance of developing postpartum depression.

Managing Postpartum Depression

Managing postpartum depression often entails a mix of various therapies, according to the individual's circumstances. Here are some popular strategies:

- Therapy: Psychotherapy, such as cognitive-behavioral therapy (CBT) or interpersonal therapy (IPT), may help people examine their emotions, develop coping techniques, and enhance their general well-being.

- Medication: In certain circumstances, healthcare providers may offer antidepressant medication to assist ease symptoms. It's crucial to talk with a healthcare practitioner to consider the risks and advantages of medicine, particularly while nursing.

- Social support: Building a solid support network is vital. This might entail requesting aid from loved ones, joining support groups, or attending postpartum support programs.

- Self-care: Prioritizing self-care activities, such as obtaining adequate rest, eating a balanced diet, participating in physical exercise, and having time for personal interests, may considerably increase well-being.

- Rest and sleep: Ensuring proper rest and sleep is vital for controlling postpartum depression. Partners, family members, or friends may give support with baby care, enabling the person to prioritize self-restoration.

- Open communication: Sharing thoughts and concerns with a trusted healthcare practitioner, spouse, or support group may bring emotional relief and help the development of successful coping skills.

Family Planning Methods and Their Importance

Family planning refers to the purposeful decision-making process regarding when to have children, how many to have, and the spacing between pregnancies. It comprises adopting numerous strategies to avoid or obtain pregnancy according to individual choices and circumstances. Here are some typical family planning methods:

Contraceptives: This category covers techniques including birth control tablets, patches, injections, implants, intrauterine devices (IUDs), and barrier methods such as condoms or diaphragms. These treatments assist prevent pregnancy by either suppressing ovulation, stopping sperm from accessing the egg or building a barrier between the sperm and egg.

Natural Techniques: Natural family planning methods entail observing fertility markers, such as menstrual cycles, basal body temperature, or cervical mucus, to determine fertile and infertile times. These approaches need careful monitoring and abstinence or the use of barrier devices during reproductive times.

Sterilization: This permanent approach includes surgical treatments like tubal ligation for women and vasectomy for males. Sterilization offers long-term contraception by blocking or severing the fallopian tubes or vas deferens, preventing sperm from reaching the egg.

Family planning is significant for various reasons

1. **Pregnancy spacing:** Adequate spacing between pregnancies helps people to recuperate physically and emotionally from the previous pregnancy and

delivery. It may lower the chance of problems for both the parent and the baby.

2. **Personal and financial considerations:** Family planning allows people the opportunity to plan and attain their desired family size, taking into account personal, financial, and professional objectives. It helps people to make educated choices about when to have children and ensures that they are ready to offer the required care and support.

3. **Health benefits:** Family planning techniques may help avoid unplanned births, which may be linked with greater risks of mother and newborn morbidity and death. They also give protection against sexually transmitted infections (STIs) when worn in combination with barrier techniques like condoms.

4. **Empowerment and autonomy:** Family planning encourages people to take control of their reproductive health and make choices that accord

with their beliefs, preferences, and circumstances. It fosters autonomy and empowers people to make educated choices about their bodies and lives.

It's crucial to remember that family planning techniques vary in terms of efficacy, side effects, and compatibility for various persons. It's advisable to speak with a healthcare physician or a family planning clinic to review the various alternatives and pick the technique that best matches your requirements and preferences.

Different family planning techniques might have varied side effects and hazards. Here are some frequent side effects or hazards connected with specific family planning methods:

Hormonal Contraceptives (Birth control pills, patches, injections, implants):

- Possible side effects: Nausea, breast discomfort, changes in menstrual flow (lighter or irregular cycles), mood fluctuations, weight gain, headaches.
- Rare risks: Increased risk of blood clots, especially in women who smoke, are overweight, or have a history of blood clots.

Intrauterine Devices (IUDs):

- Common side effects: Cramping and pain during and after insertion, irregular bleeding or spotting between periods for the first several months, and backaches.

- Rare risks: Perforation of the uterus after insertion (rare), higher risk of pelvic inflammatory disease (PID) during the first few weeks following insertion (rare).

Barrier Methods (Condoms, diaphragms):

- Possible adverse effects: Allergic responses to latex or other materials, diminished sensitivity during intercourse.
- Risks: Condoms may break or come off if not used properly, which can result in pregnancy or possible exposure to sexually transmitted diseases (STIs).

Natural Family Planning Methods (Tracking fertility signs):

- Possible adverse effects: Requires frequent and precise surveillance of fertility indications, which may be tough and time-consuming. It may also entail periods of abstinence or the use of barrier techniques during fertile seasons.
- Risks: Higher chance of unexpected pregnancy compared to other family planning techniques if not followed appropriately or if fertility indications are misread.

Sterilization (Tubal ligation for women, vasectomy for men):

- Common side effects: Soreness and discomfort at the location of the surgery, transient alterations in monthly bleeding for women.

- Uncommon risks: Risk of surgical complications, failure or reversal of the surgery (albeit uncommon), regret or unhappiness with the irreversible nature of sterilization.

It's vital to remember that the side effects and hazards might differ based on individual circumstances, such as general health, medical history, and lifestyle. It's advisable to speak with a healthcare professional or a family planning clinic to review the unique side effects and dangers linked with various procedures and to pick the most suited approach depending on your requirements and circumstances.

Additionally, it's worth highlighting that certain family planning techniques, such as hormonal contraceptives, may have additional advantages beyond contraception, such as lowering the chance of certain health disorders including ovarian cysts, endometrial cancer, and pelvic inflammatory disease. However, it's crucial to examine these possible advantages and hazards with a healthcare expert to make an educated choice.

Remember that family planning techniques should be selected based on individual choices, medical concerns, and consultations with healthcare specialists.

CONCLUSION

In "Pregnancy Compass: Everything you need to know about your baby's growth and development, your body changes, and your Prenatal care options," we have examined a plethora of material to aid you through this changing journey. Let's outline the important elements and insights that will empower you with information, confidence, and a better understanding of pregnancy.

Main Points and Takeaways

1. Baby's Growth and Development: We have dived into the remarkable journey of your baby's growth and development, from conception to delivery. Understanding the many phases and milestones

might help you connect with the marvel of life developing inside you.

2. Your Body Changes: Pregnancy brings about considerable changes in your body. We have explored the physical and hormonal alterations you might anticipate, giving insights and recommendations to overcome typical discomforts and appreciate the beauty of this changing time.

3. Prenatal Care Options: Prenatal care is crucial for the health and well-being of both you and your baby. We have covered numerous prenatal care alternatives, stressing the significance of frequent check-ups, tests, and consultations with healthcare specialists to ensure a safe pregnancy.

4. Empowerment and Decision-Making: Throughout the book, we have highlighted the significance of empowerment and informed decision-making. By providing you with thorough information, we seek to enable you to make decisions that match your beliefs, tastes, and particular circumstances.

In "Pregnancy Compass," we have endeavoured to present you with a brief but informative and compelling guide to navigate the complicated and awe-inspiring adventure of pregnancy. We hope this book has provided you with the information and courage to make educated choices, love the wondrous changes occurring inside you, and embrace the pleasure of being a parent.

Thank you for picking "Pregnancy Compass" as your companion on this incredible trip. We wish you a healthy and memorable pregnancy journey filled with love, excitement, and anticipation for the glorious chapter of motherhood ahead.

Congratulations on finishing your pregnancy adventure! You have begun a beautiful experience of motherhood. We would love to know your opinion and experience with this book. Your helpful feedback can help us improve.

Final Tips and Advice on Parenting and Motherhood

1. Prioritize Self-Care: As a parent, it's vital to prioritize self-care. Take time for yourself, indulge in things that offer you pleasure and relaxation, and

seek help from loved ones or professional resources when required. Remember, taking care of yourself helps you to be the best parent you can be.

2. Build a Support Network: Surround yourself with a supportive network of family, friends, and other parents. Share your experiences, get advice, and depend on one another throughout the ups and downs of motherhood. Having a support system may give emotional affirmation, direction, and a feeling of belonging.

3. Trust Your Instincts: Motherhood comes with a variety of advice and views, but remember that you know your kid best. Trust your instincts and make judgements that correspond with your ideals and intuition. You are the authority on your child's needs and well-being.

4. Embrace Imperfection: Parenthood is a journey filled with highs and lows. Embrace the faults and recognise that it's normal to make errors. Learn from them, forgive yourself, and concentrate on the love and connection you have with your kid.

5. Cultivate open conversation: As your kid develops, cultivate open and polite conversation. Create a secure atmosphere where your youngster feels comfortable sharing their ideas and feelings. Listen intently, acknowledge their emotions, and participate in meaningful discussions to create trust and understanding.

Thank you for selecting this book as your guide through pregnancy, postpartum, and beyond. We congratulate you on finishing your pregnancy journey and wish you a successful and joyous experience as a parent.

Wishing you love, strength, and happiness in your parenting experience.

Sincerely,

Harbbie Yeenks

www.ingramcontent.com/pod-product-compliance
Lightning Source LLC
Chambersburg PA
CBHW061646250726
48659CB00004B/1389